I0701781

Unmasking the Silent Killer:

Chronic Wasting Disease and its Menace on Wildlife

DR VICTORIA WILDWOOD

Copyright © 2023 Dr Victoria Wildwood

All rights reserved. No part of this book may be reproduced or transmitted in any form or by any means, electronic or mechanical, including photocopying, recording or by any information storage and retrieval system, without written permission from the author.

Table of contents…………..

ABOUT DR VICTORIA WILDWOOD

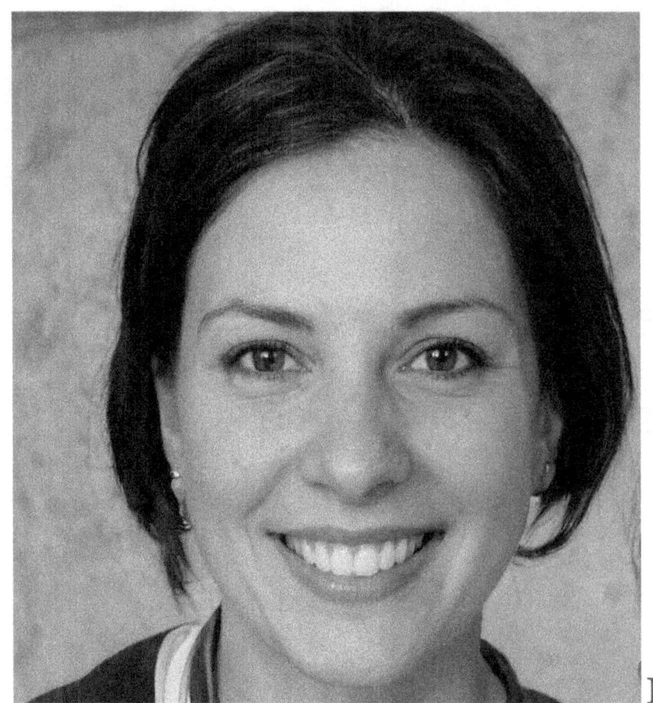

In the small town of Everwood, nestled on the edge of a vast and mysterious forest, lived the renowned wildlife disease specialist, Dr. Victoria Wildwood. Dr. Wildwood wasn't just a doctor; she was a guardian of the natural world, a tireless advocate for the health of the forest's inhabitants. Known for her unwavering dedication to understanding and combating the enigmatic Chronic Wasting Disease, Dr. Wildwood had earned a reputation that echoed through the dense woods and quiet streams of Everwood. The townsfolk spoke of her with a mix of awe and gratitude, for she had become a symbol of hope in the face of an invisible threat that loomed over their beloved wildlife.

INTRODUCTION TO THE CHRONIC WASTING DISEASE

Chronic Wasting Disease (CWD) is a progressive and fatal neurological disease that affects cervids, which are members of the deer family. This disease primarily impacts deer, elk, reindeer, and moose. CWD belongs to a group of diseases known as transmissible spongiform encephalopathies (TSEs), which also includes diseases like mad cow disease in cattle and Creutzfeldt-Jakob disease in humans.

In the heart of Everwood, where whispers of the ancient forest carried tales of mystery and magic, there lived a luminary whose name echoed through the dense canopy like a secret incantation — Dr. Victoria

Wildwood. Her story, a symphony of science and wilderness, unfolds like a tapestry woven with threads of dedication, curiosity, and an unwavering commitment to the delicate dance of nature.

As dawn painted the treetops in hues of gold, and dusk descended with a symphony of night creatures, Dr. Wildwood emerged as the guardian of this enchanted realm. In the pages that follow, prepare to embark on a journey into the heart of Everwood, where the fate of its majestic inhabitants hangs in the balance.

The air crackles with anticipation as Chronic Wasting Disease, a silent spectre haunting the shadows, threatens to unravel the very fabric of this wild tapestry. Enter the world of Dr. Victoria Wildwood, a virtuoso of veterinary science, a whisperer to the creatures of the forest, and a luminary on a quest to decipher the enigma of an elusive and perilous foe.

In the small town at the edge of the woods, where the ordinary and the extraordinary converge, Dr. Wildwood's tale begins. It is a tale of tireless research beneath the emerald canopy, of a scientist's dance with the unknown, and of a healer's communion with the spirit of the wild.

Buckle your seatbelts, for this is not just a journey into the intricacies of Chronic Wasting Disease; it is an odyssey into the soul of a dedicated guardian, a saga of nature's resilience, and a testament to the extraordinary connection between humankind and the untamed world. As we venture forth into the realms of Everwood, let Dr. Victoria Wildwood guides us through the pages of a captivating story that transcends the boundaries of science and plunges us deep into the heart of an untamed, awe-inspiring wilderness.

Here are some key points about Chronic Wasting Disease

Etiology and Transmission:

CWD is caused by abnormal proteins called prions, which affect the brain and nervous system of infected animals.

The disease is transmitted horizontally, meaning it can be spread directly between animals through contact with saliva, urine, feces, and other bodily fluids.

Geographical Distribution:

CWD has been identified in various regions of North America, including the United States and Canada.

The disease has also been reported in other parts of the world, albeit to a lesser extent.

Symptoms:

Clinical signs of CWD include weight loss, excessive salivation, stumbling, lack of coordination, and changes in behavior.

Infected animals may exhibit a vacant stare and may be found in poor body condition.

Impact on Wildlife Management:

CWD poses significant challenges for wildlife management and conservation efforts, as infected populations can experience declines.

The disease has implications for the hunting industry and can impact the health of wild cervid populations.

Research and Surveillance:

Scientists and wildlife agencies conduct research to better understand the transmission, prevalence, and impact of CWD.

Surveillance programs are implemented to monitor the spread of the disease and to identify infected individuals.

Preventive Measures:

Due to the lack of a cure or effective treatment for CWD, prevention is a key focus.

Measures such as restrictions on the movement of deer and elk, culling infected individuals, and public education campaigns are implemented to manage the disease.

Human Health Concerns:

While there is no conclusive evidence that CWD can infect humans, it is recommended to avoid consuming meat from infected animals as a precaution.

Challenges and Controversies:

The management of CWD is a complex issue, and there are debates about the most effective strategies for controlling its spread.

Balancing wildlife conservation and disease management efforts is a persistent challenge.

Addressing the complexities of Chronic Wasting Disease requires a multi-faceted approach that involves research, surveillance, and cooperation among wildlife agencies, scientists, and the public. Ongoing efforts are essential to mitigate the impact of CWD on cervid populations and maintain the overall health of ecosystems.

Research Efforts:

Ongoing research is crucial for understanding the biology of the prions responsible for CWD and developing effective strategies for diagnosis and management.

Scientists are studying the genetic factors that may contribute to susceptibility or resistance to the disease among cervid populations.

Diagnostic Techniques:

Accurate and early detection of CWD is essential for implementing effective management strategies.

Advances in diagnostic techniques, including post-mortem tests and live animal testing, are areas of active research.

Interactions with Other Species:

Understanding the potential for CWD transmission to other animal species is a topic of concern.

Research is ongoing to determine if there are risks associated with the consumption of plants grown in areas inhabited by infected cervids.

Public Awareness and Education:

Public education campaigns are critical to raise awareness about CWD and promote responsible practices among hunters, wildlife enthusiasts, and the general public.

Clear communication about the risks and preventive measures can help in minimizing the spread of the disease.

International Collaboration:

Given the potential for the spread of CWD across borders, international collaboration is essential.

Wildlife management agencies, researchers, and policymakers from different countries share information and strategies to collectively address the challenges posed by CWD.

Ethical Considerations:

The culling of infected animals as a management strategy raises ethical considerations.

Striking a balance between controlling the spread of the disease and respecting the rights of wildlife is an ongoing debate.

Long-Term Ecosystem Effects:

The long-term ecological impact of CWD on ecosystems, including changes in vegetation and interactions with other species, is an area of ongoing study.

Understanding how CWD may alter the dynamics of wildlife populations and ecosystems is crucial for effective management.

Development of Vaccines or Treatments:

The development of vaccines or treatments for CWD remains a significant goal for researchers.

Progress in this area could offer new tools for managing and potentially eradicating the disease.

Chronic Wasting Disease presents a complex and evolving challenge for wildlife management and conservation. Ongoing scientific research, effective surveillance programs, and international cooperation are essential components of a comprehensive strategy to address the impacts of CWD on cervid populations and ecosystems. As our understanding of the disease deepens, it is likely that new insights and innovative approaches will continue to shape the management and mitigation of Chronic Wasting Disease in the future.

HOW TO PREVENT IT

Preventing the spread of Chronic Wasting Disease (CWD) involves a combination of management strategies, regulations, and public awareness. Here are some key measures that can be taken to help prevent and control CWD:

Surveillance and Monitoring:

> Implement robust surveillance programs to monitor the prevalence of CWD in wild cervid populations.

> Conduct regular testing of harvested animals, especially in regions where CWD has been detected.

Movement Restrictions:

> Enforce restrictions on the movement of captive cervids to prevent the spread of CWD.

Regulate the transportation of live animals and their body parts to minimize the risk of introducing the disease to new areas.

Culling Infected Individuals:

Implement targeted culling of infected individuals in affected populations to reduce the spread of the disease.

This strategy aims to lower the density of infected animals, decreasing the likelihood of transmission.

Decontamination and Biosecurity:

Establish and promote biosecurity measures in captive cervid facilities to prevent the introduction and transmission of CWD.

Implement measures such as cleaning and disinfecting equipment and facilities to minimize the risk of contamination.

Hunting Regulations:

Adjust hunting regulations to manage and control deer populations in areas affected by CWD.

Consider changes to hunting seasons, bag limits, and other regulations to help control the spread of the disease.

Public Education:

Raise awareness among hunters, wildlife enthusiasts, and the general public about CWD and its transmission risks.

Promote responsible practices, such as proper disposal of carcasses and reporting of sick animals.

Avoid Feeding Wildlife:

Discourage supplemental feeding of deer and other cervids, as concentrated feeding areas can facilitate the transmission of CWD.

Minimize the congregation of animals in specific locations to reduce the risk of disease spread.

Research and Development:

Invest in research to develop diagnostic tools, vaccines, and treatments for CWD.

Ongoing scientific efforts are essential for advancing our understanding of the disease and developing effective preventive measures.

International Collaboration:

Collaborate with neighboring regions and countries to share information, experiences, and strategies for managing and preventing CWD.

Coordinate efforts to prevent the cross-border spread of the disease.

Ethical Considerations:

Consider ethical implications when implementing management strategies, especially when culling is involved.

Engage with stakeholders, including hunters and local communities, to address concerns and ensure a balanced and ethical approach.

It's important to note that while some preventive measures are already in place, the effectiveness of these strategies may vary based on the specific circumstances in each region. Ongoing research, adaptive management, and a collaborative approach involving wildlife agencies, researchers, and the public are crucial for successfully preventing and managing Chronic Wasting Disease.

Regulation of Commercial Activities:

Monitor and regulate commercial activities involving cervids, such as game farms, to prevent the potential spread of CWD through the movement of live animals.

Traceability and Record Keeping:

Establish systems for traceability and record-keeping in the cervid farming industry to track the movement of animals and identify potential sources of infection.

Research on Prion Persistence:

Investigate the environmental persistence of prions responsible for CWD. Understanding how prions remain in the environment can inform strategies for reducing the risk of transmission.

Development of Prion-Resistant Strains:

Explore selective breeding programs aimed at developing cervid populations with increased resistance to CWD.

This could be a long-term strategy for reducing the prevalence of the disease in affected areas.

Community Engagement:

Engage local communities, hunters, and landowners in CWD management efforts.

Encourage the reporting of sick animals, and involve the community in developing and implementing prevention strategies.

International Standards and Guidelines:

Work towards the establishment of international standards and guidelines for the prevention and management of CWD.

Collaborate with international organizations to share best practices and coordinate efforts on a global scale.

Funding for Research and Management:

Allocate sufficient funding for research on CWD, including its epidemiology, transmission dynamics, and potential control measures.

Ensure that wildlife management agencies have the resources needed to implement effective control strategies.

Adaptive Management:

Embrace adaptive management approaches that allow for flexibility in strategies based on new scientific findings and changes in the distribution and prevalence of CWD.

Public-Private Partnerships:

Foster collaboration between government agencies, non-profit organizations, and the private sector to pool resources and expertise in the fight against CWD.

Early Detection and Rapid Response:

Develop and implement systems for early detection of CWD outbreaks to enable rapid response and containment efforts.

Swift action can be crucial in preventing the further spread of the disease.

Education in Schools and Training Programs:

Integrate information about CWD into school curricula and training programs for wildlife professionals.

Educating the next generation of wildlife stewards can contribute to a culture of responsible management and conservation.

Integration with Overall Ecosystem Management:

Consider CWD management within the broader context of ecosystem health and management.

Understand the interconnections between wildlife populations, vegetation, and other species to develop holistic and sustainable management strategies.

Addressing Chronic Wasting Disease requires a comprehensive and adaptive approach that takes into account the ecological, social, and economic dimensions of the issue. By combining research, regulatory measures, public engagement, and international cooperation, there is potential to minimize the impact of CWD on cervid populations and the ecosystems they inhabit.

www.ingramcontent.com/pod-product-compliance
Lightning Source LLC
Chambersburg PA
CBHW060911260726
48661CB00008B/3583